# GRAYSCALE

## COLORING BOOKS FOR BEGINNERS

VOL.2

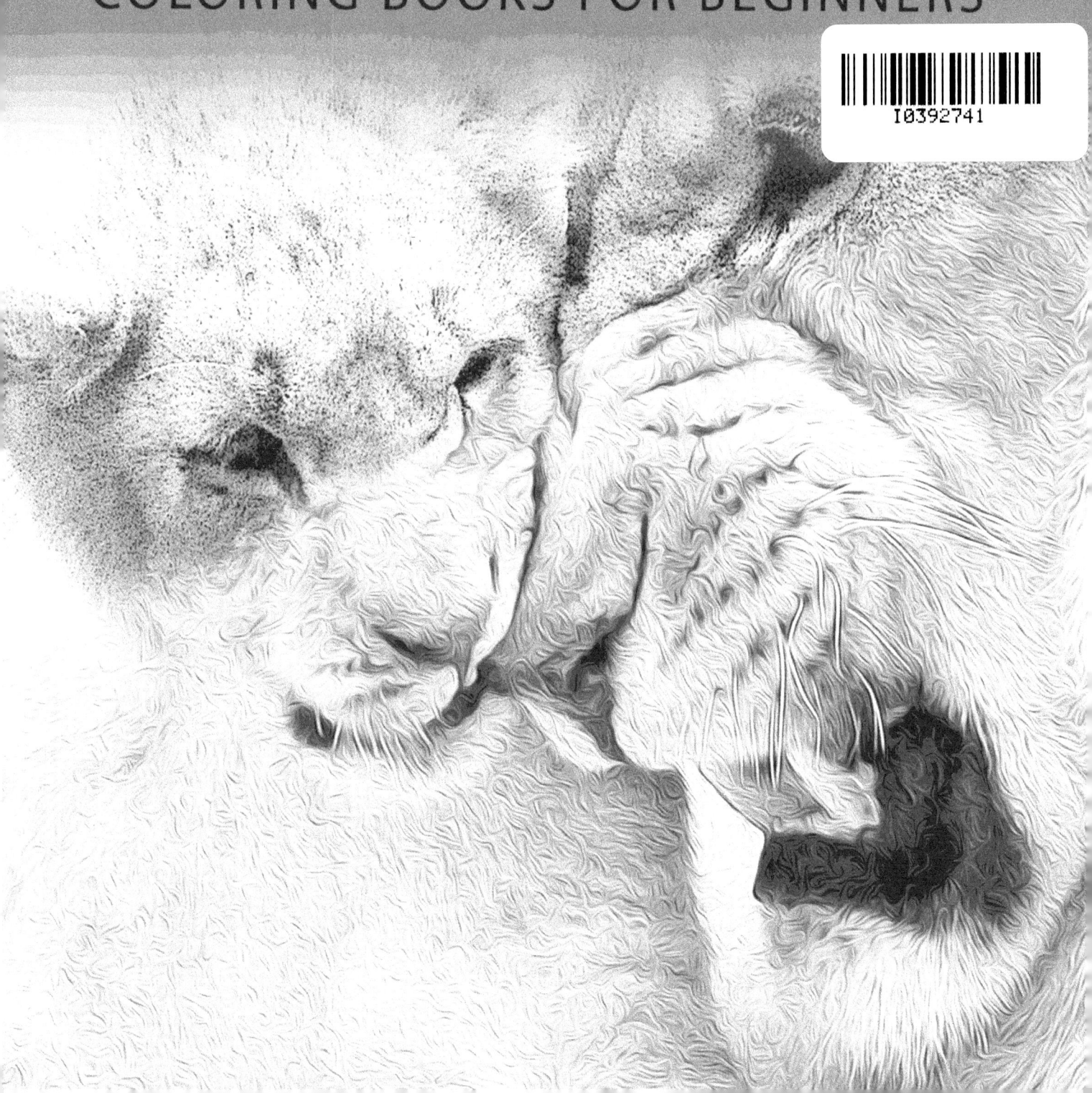

# COLOR TEST PAGE

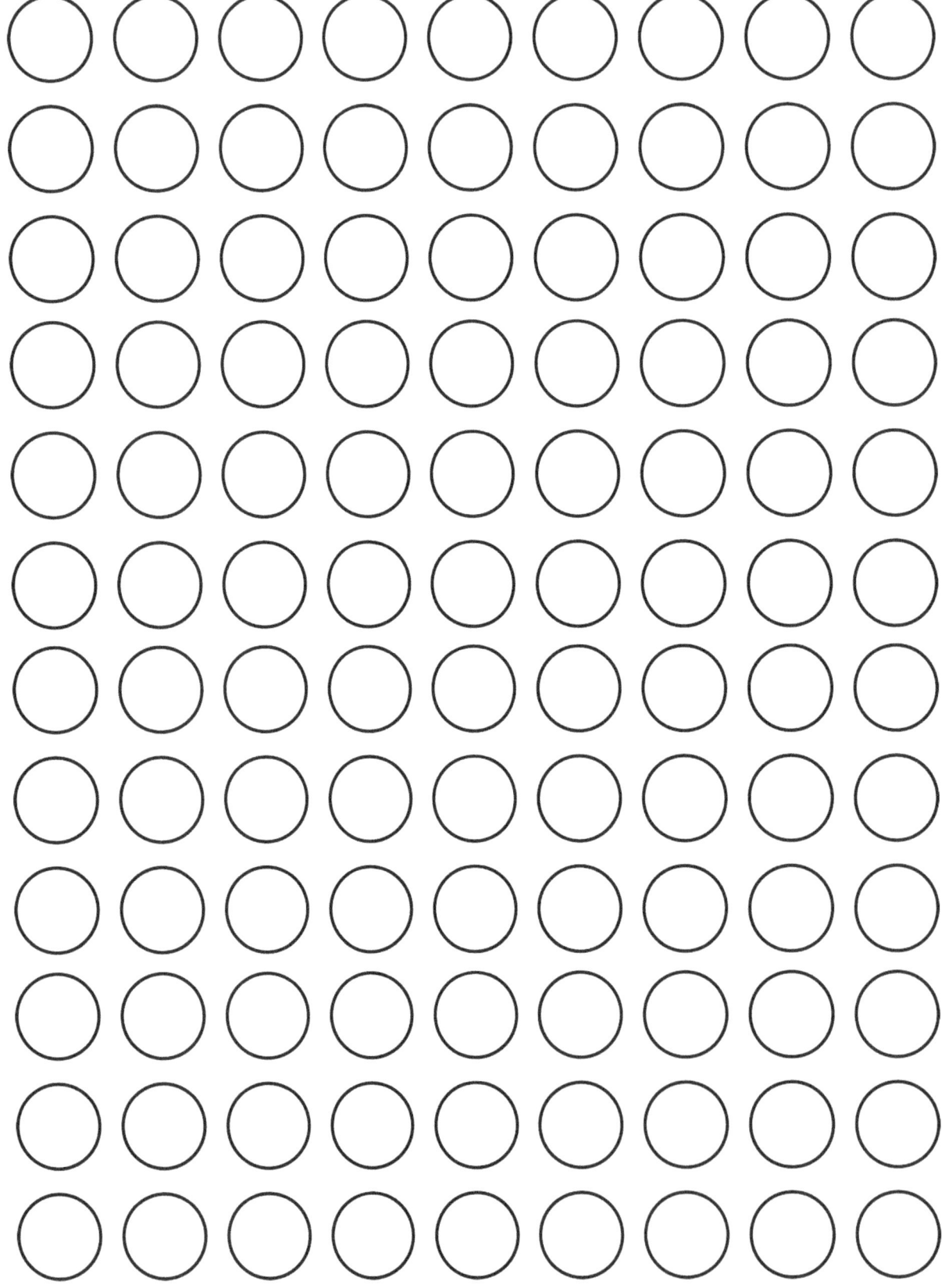

# COLOR TEST PAGE

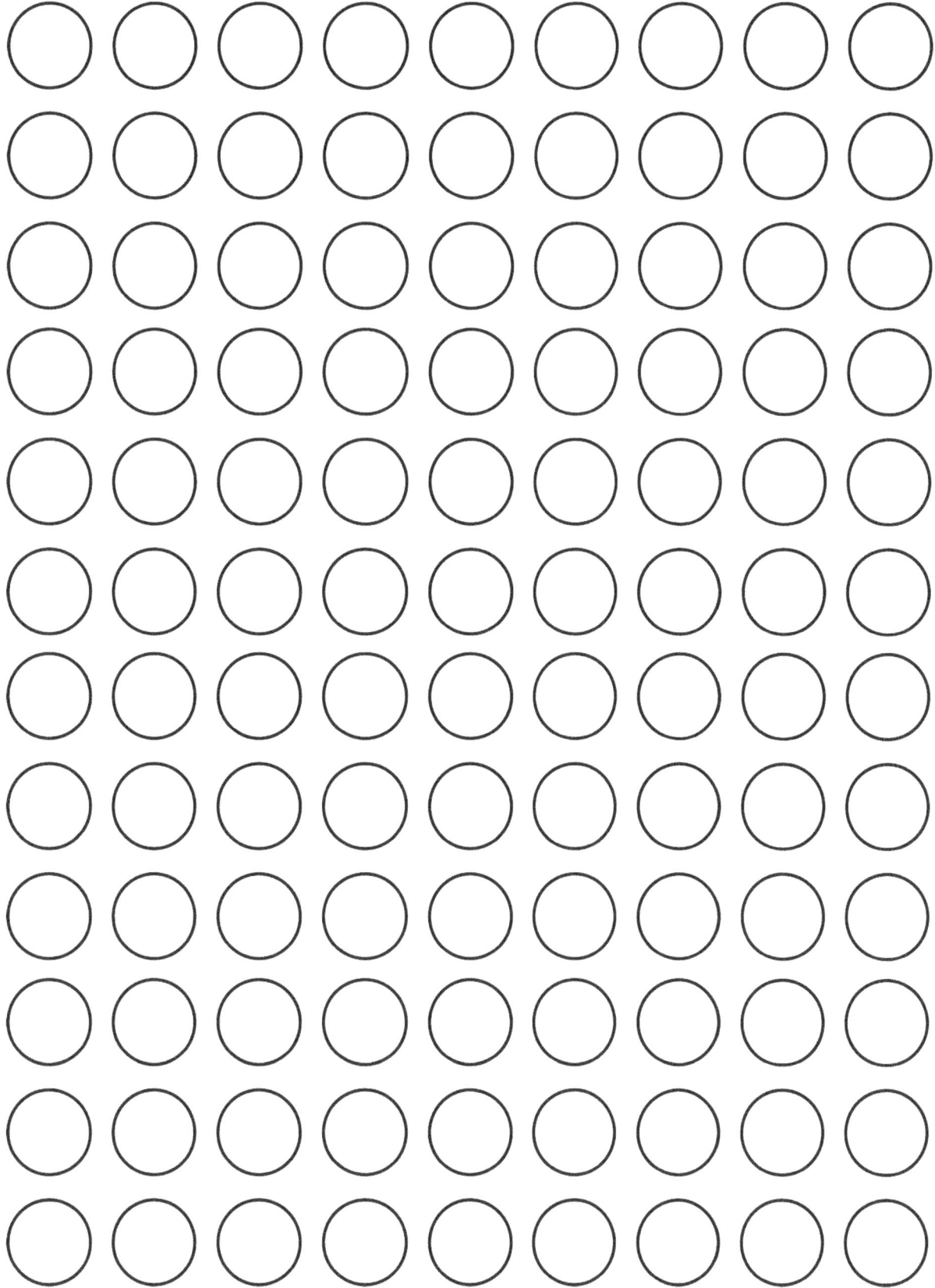

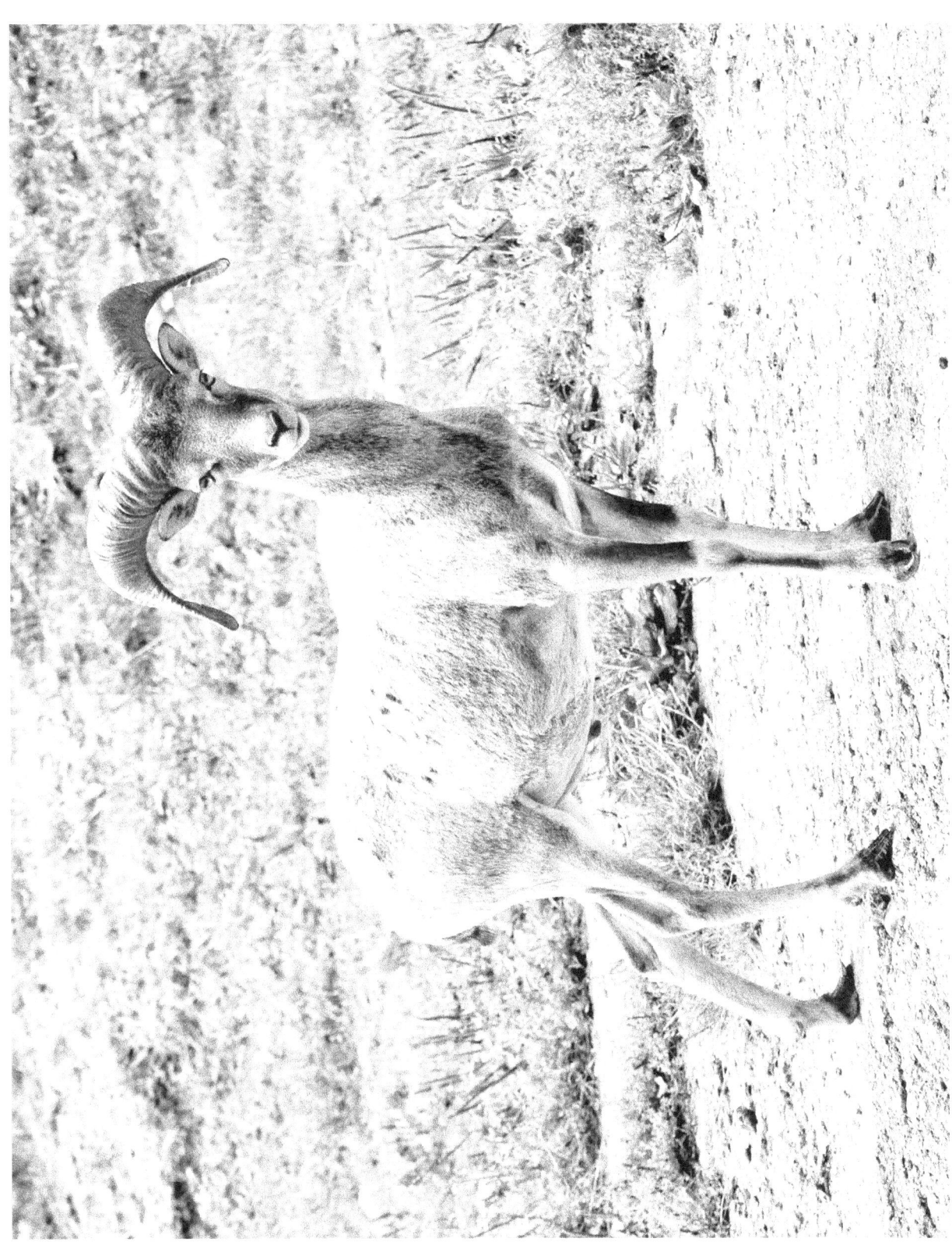

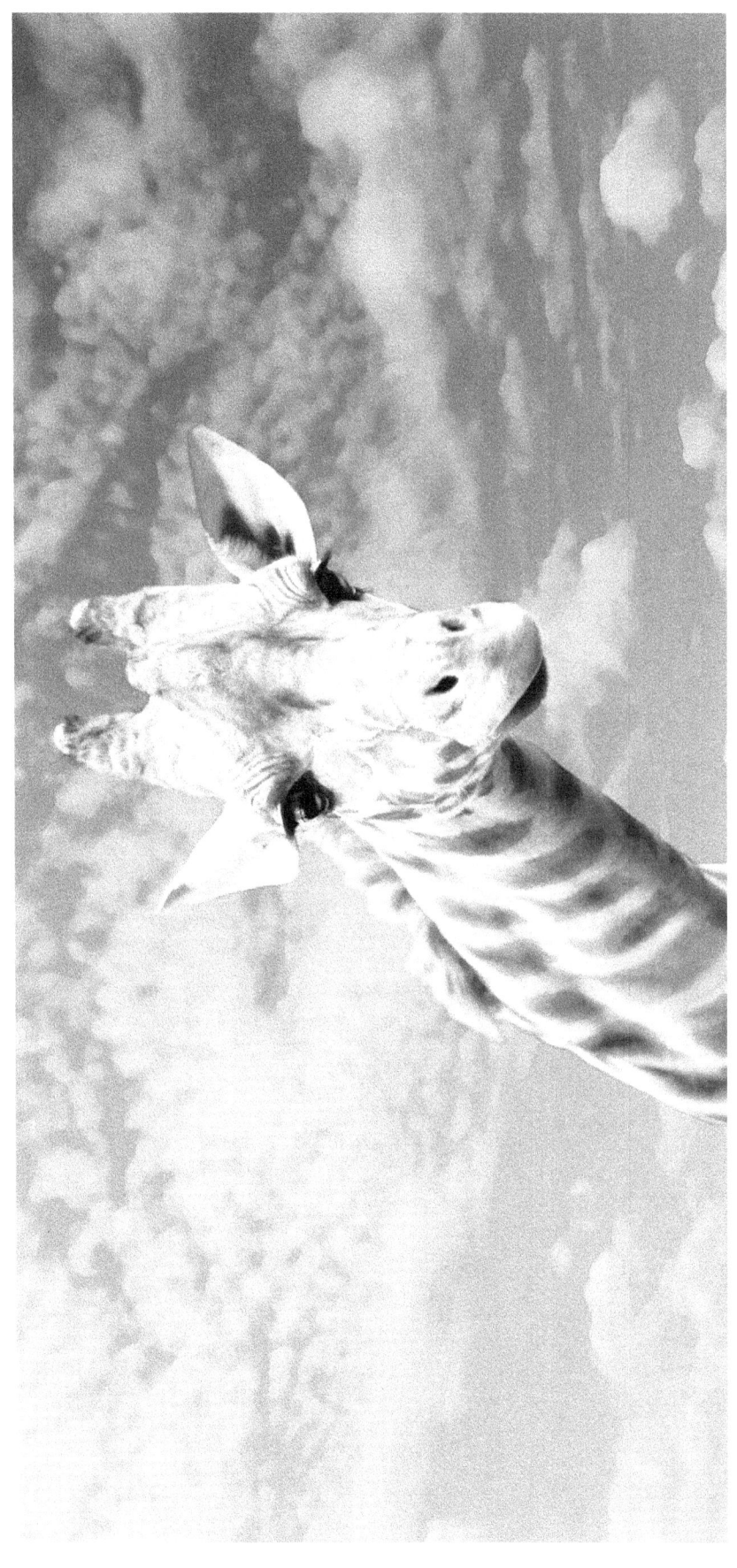

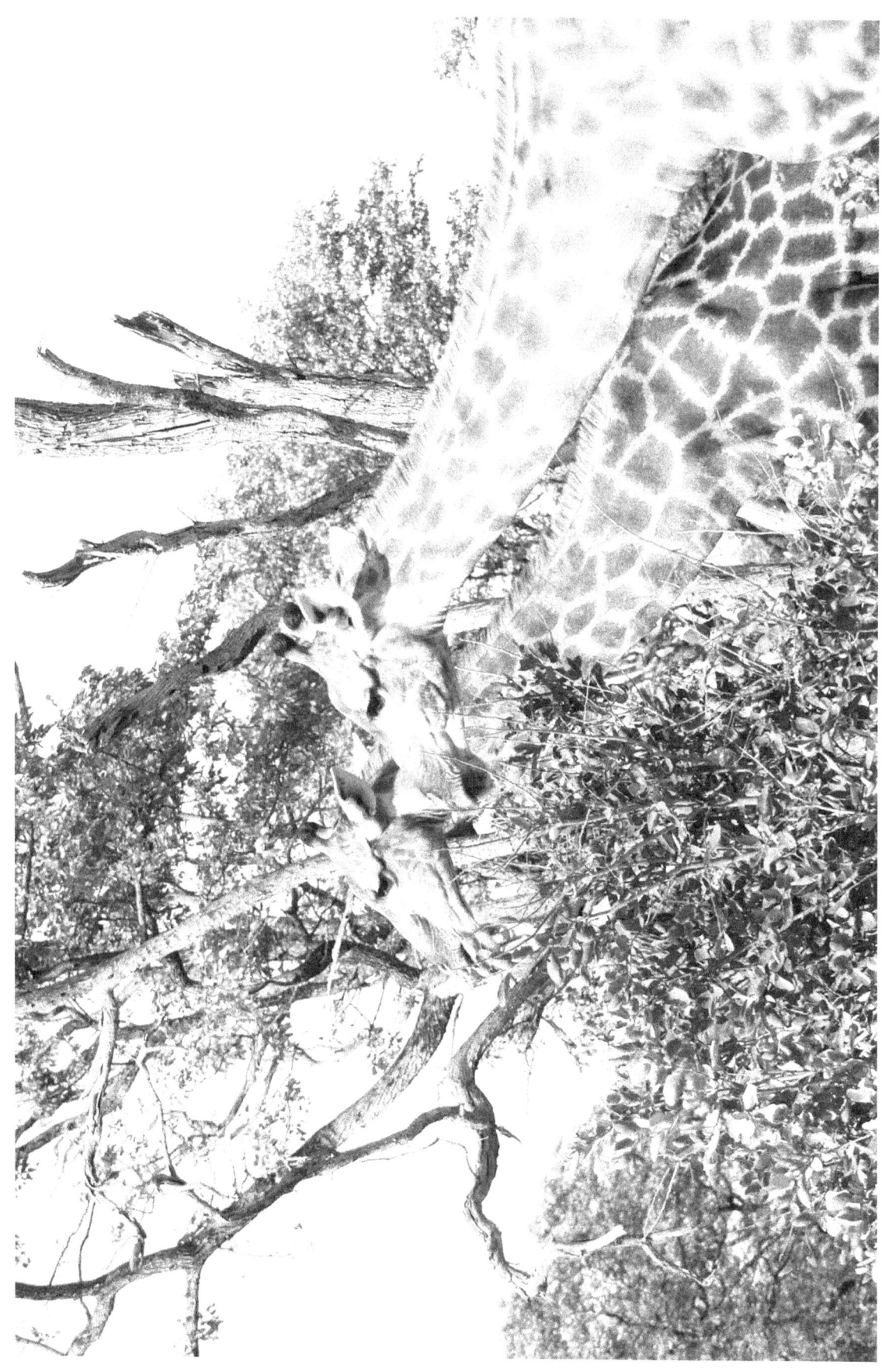

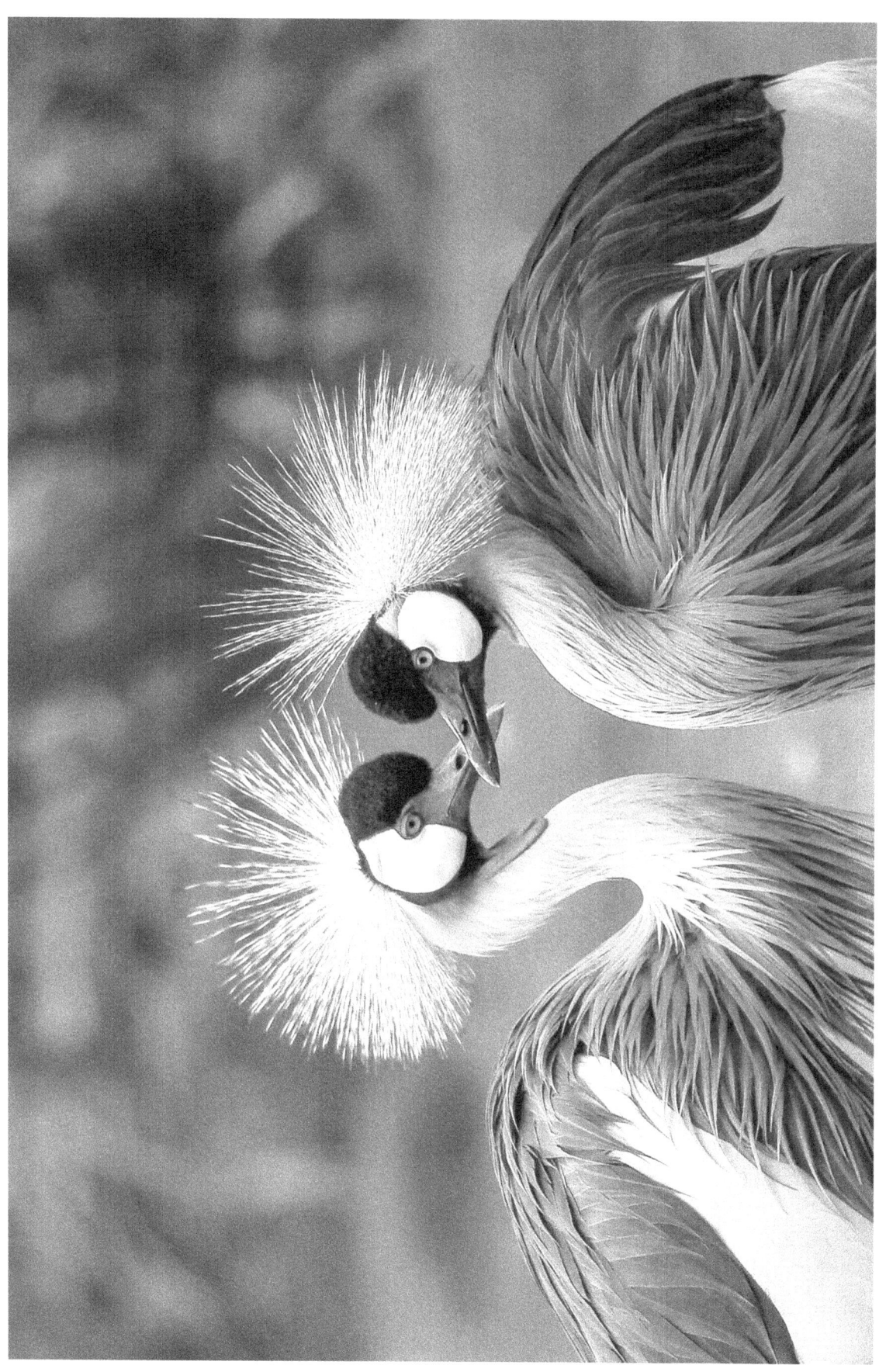

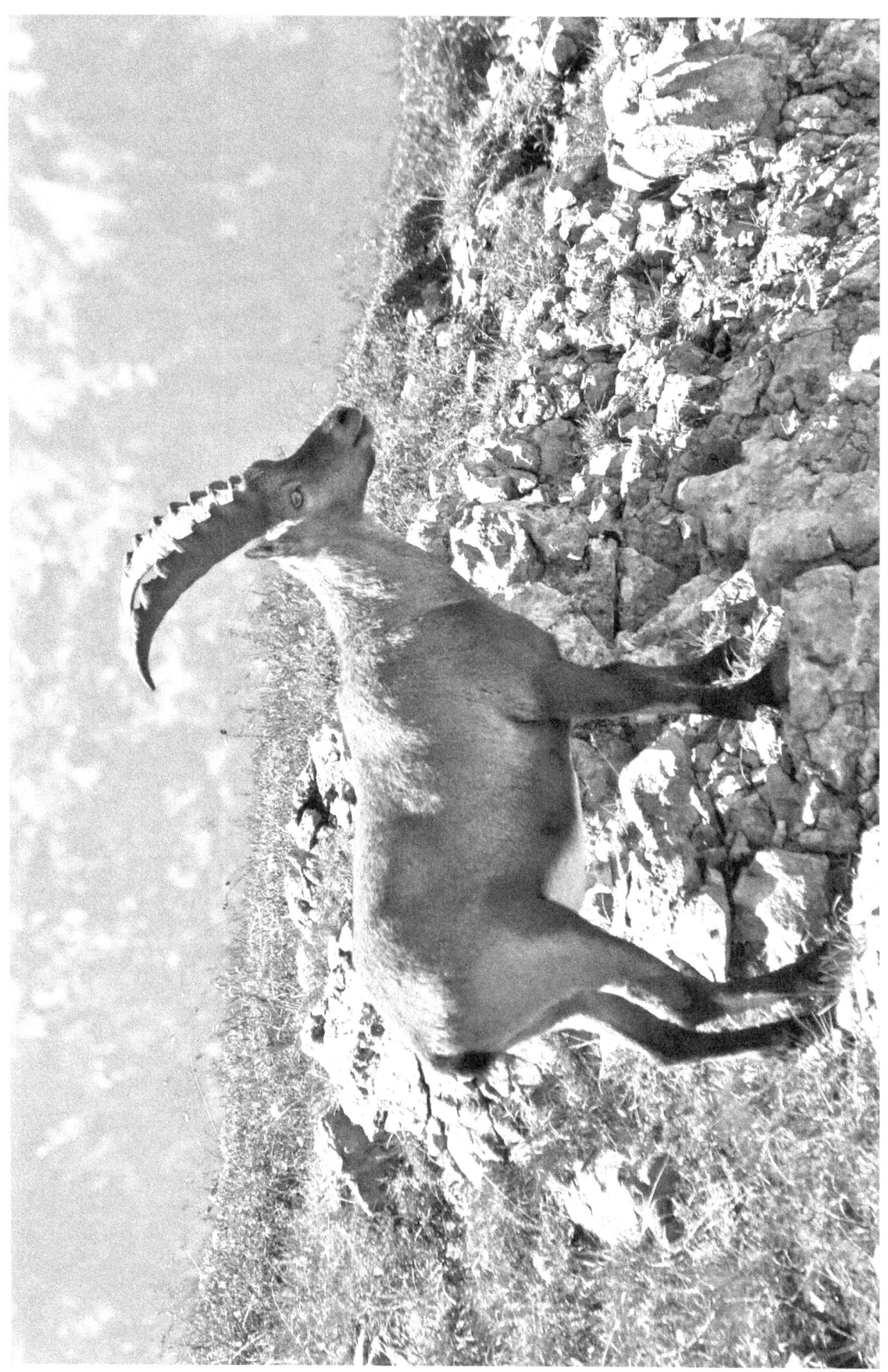

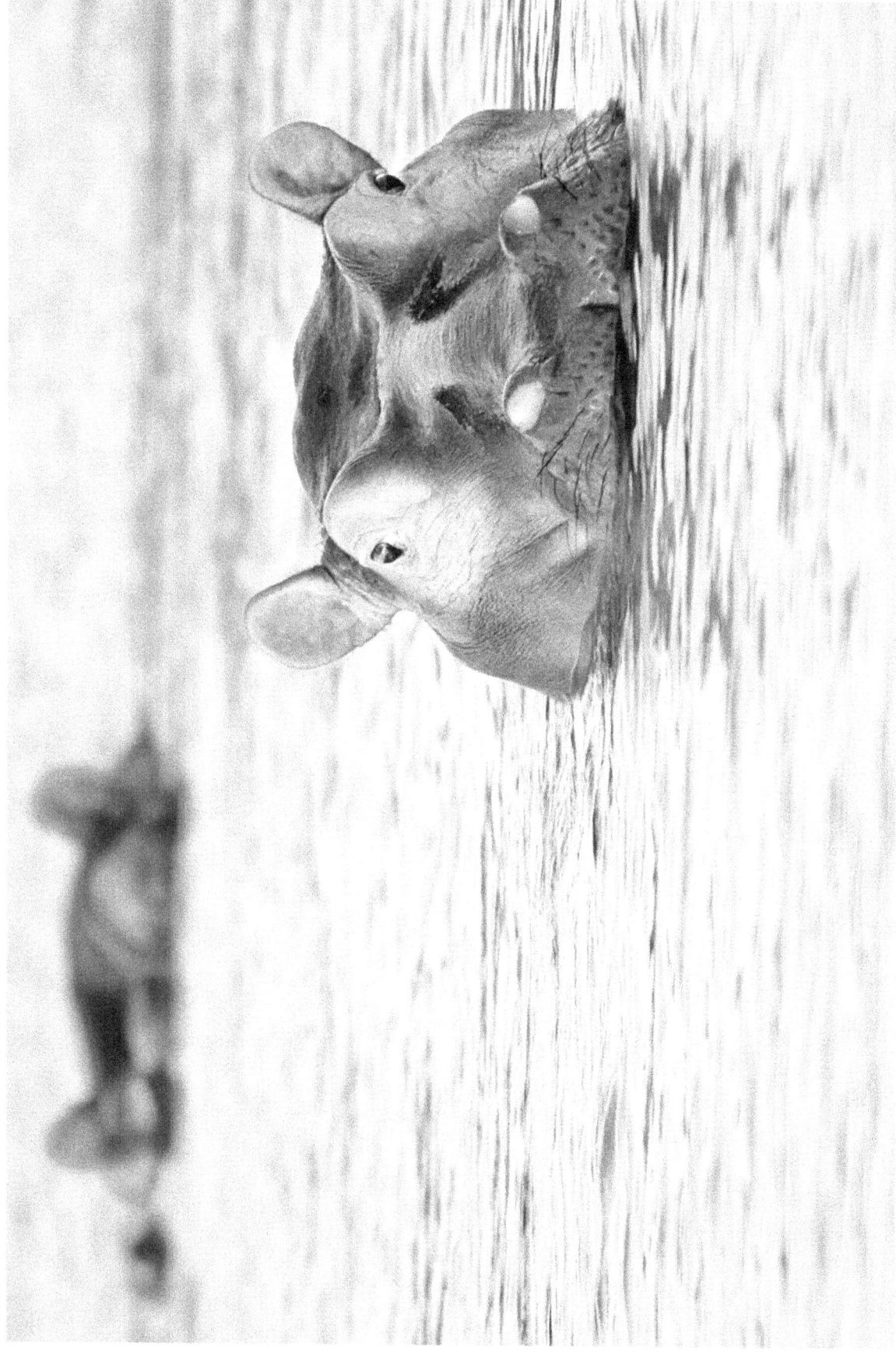

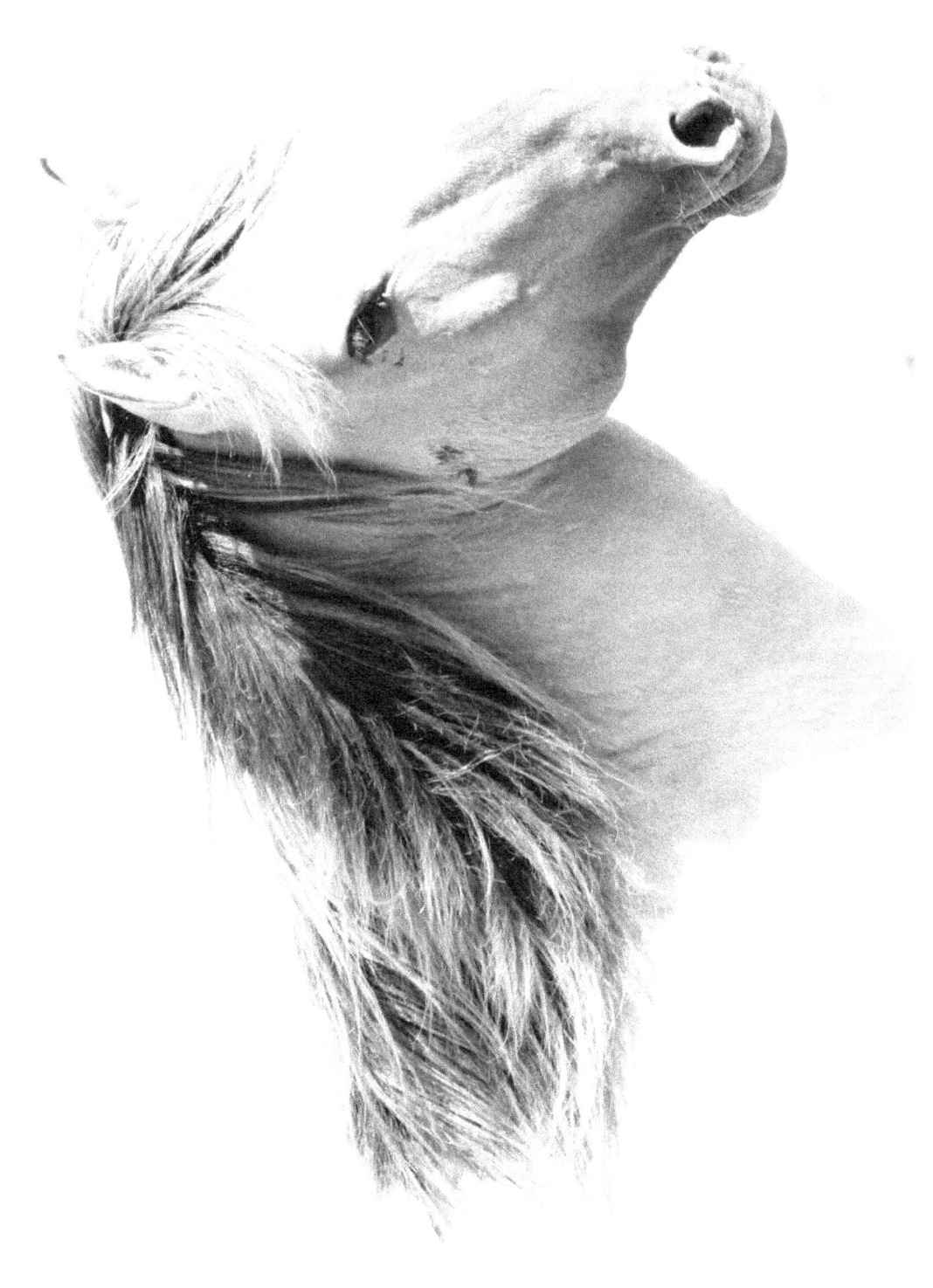

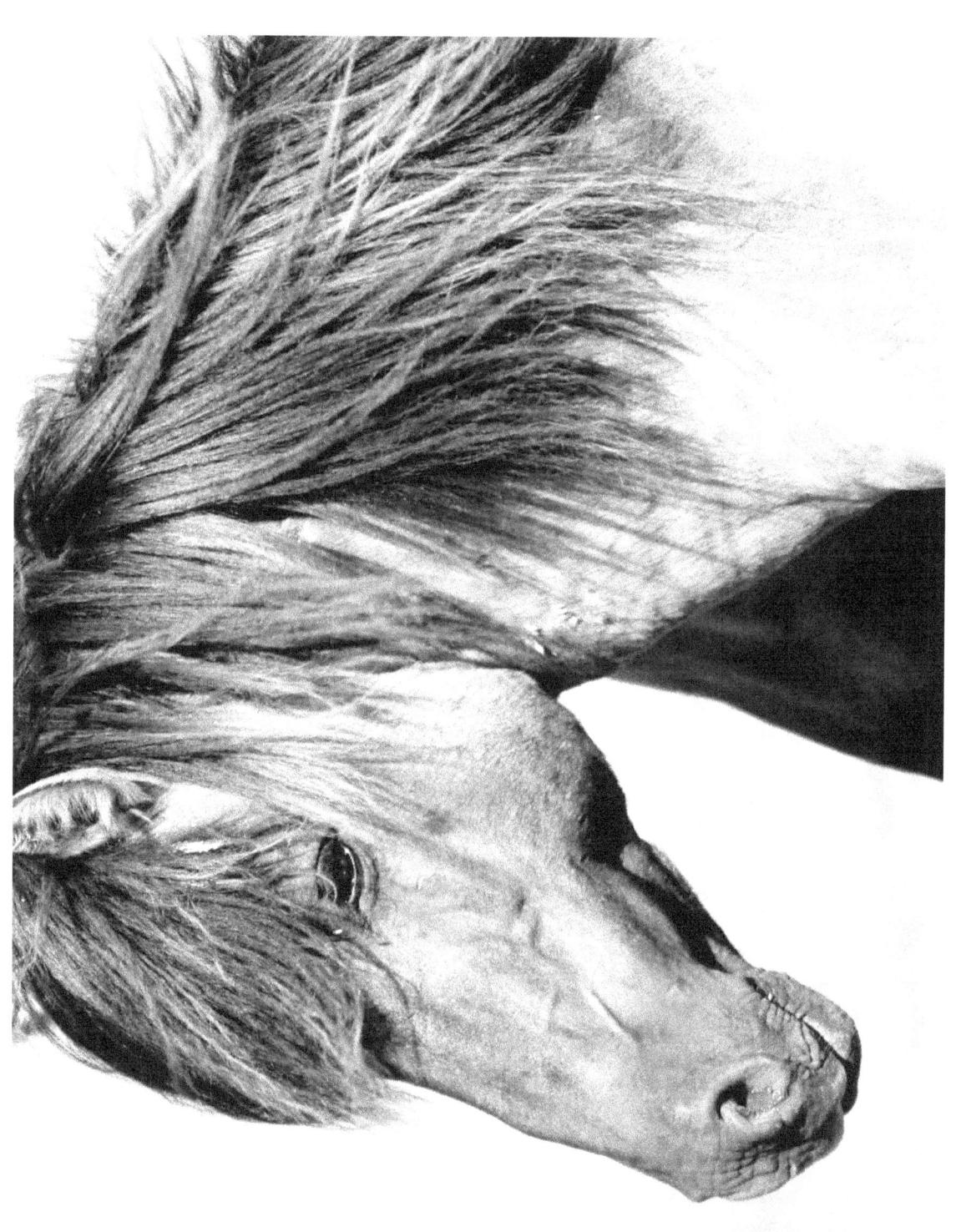

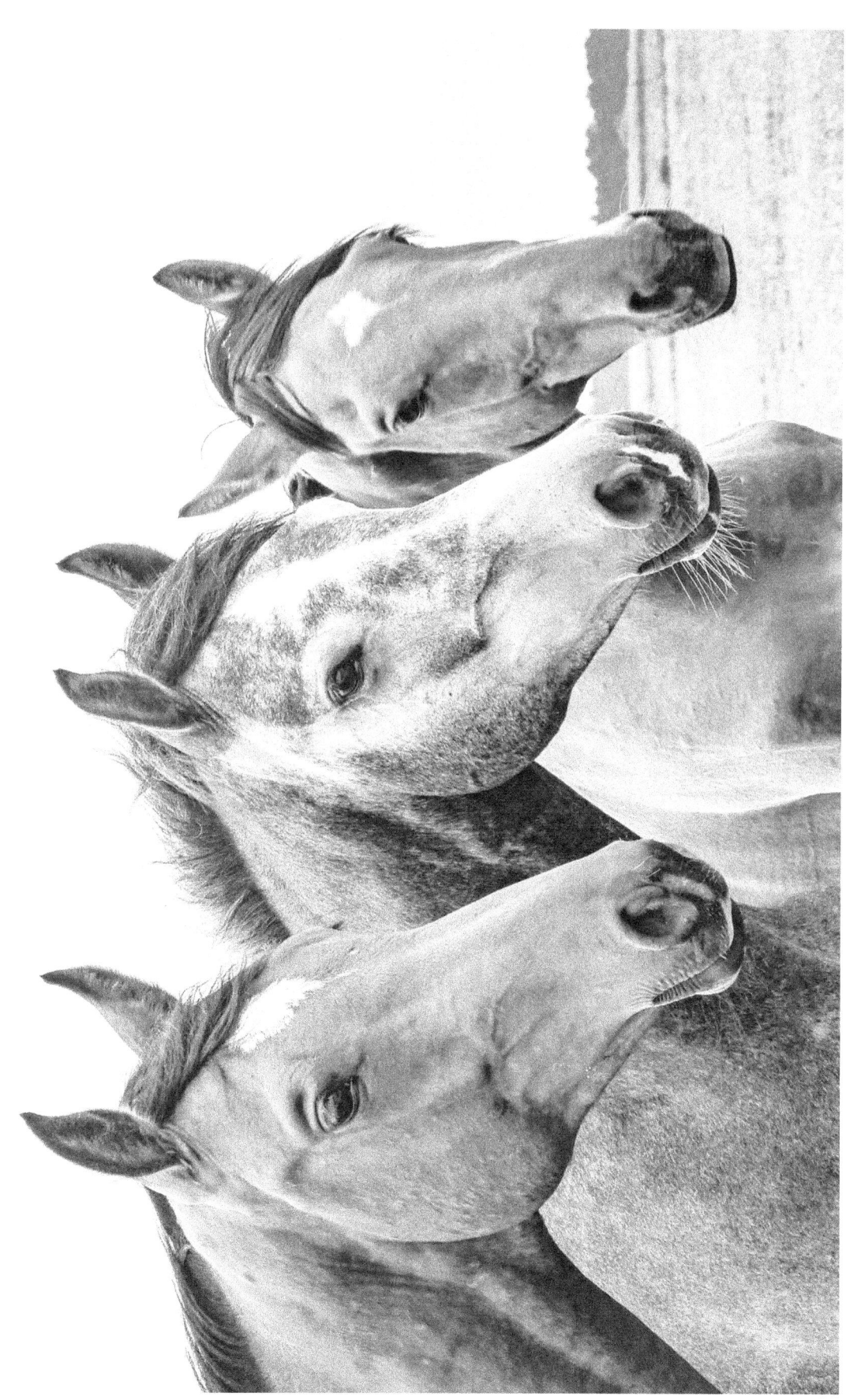

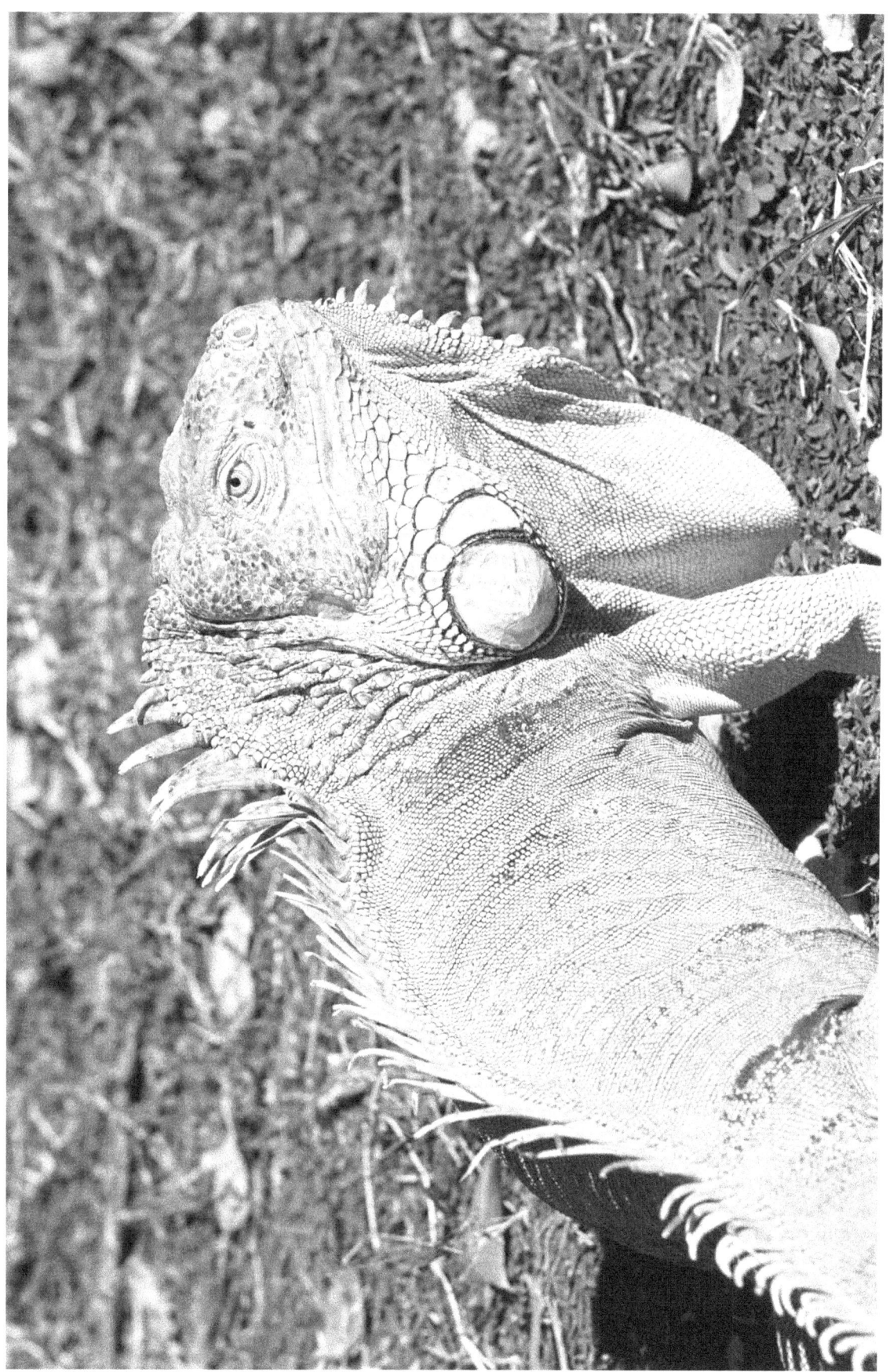

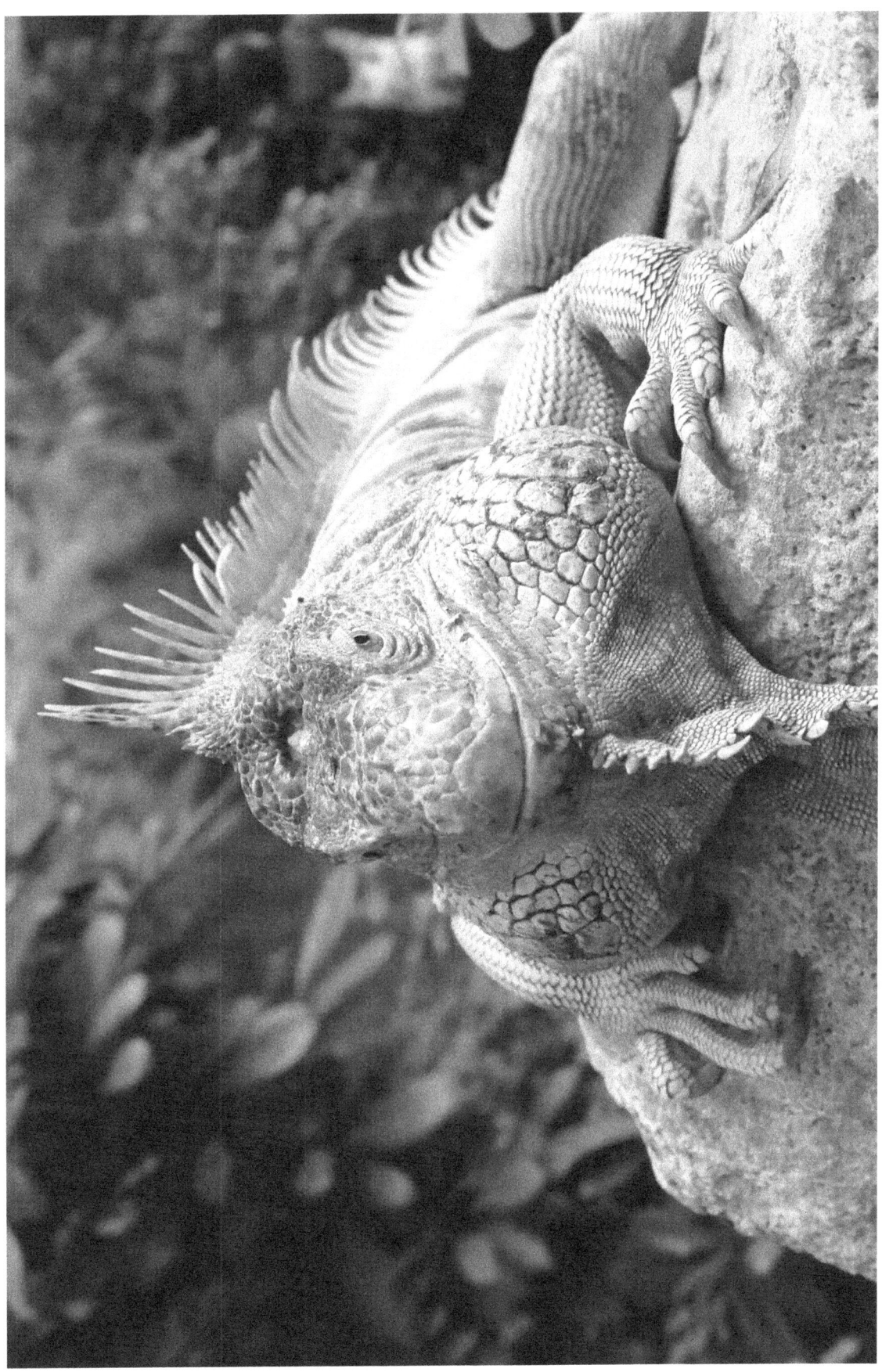

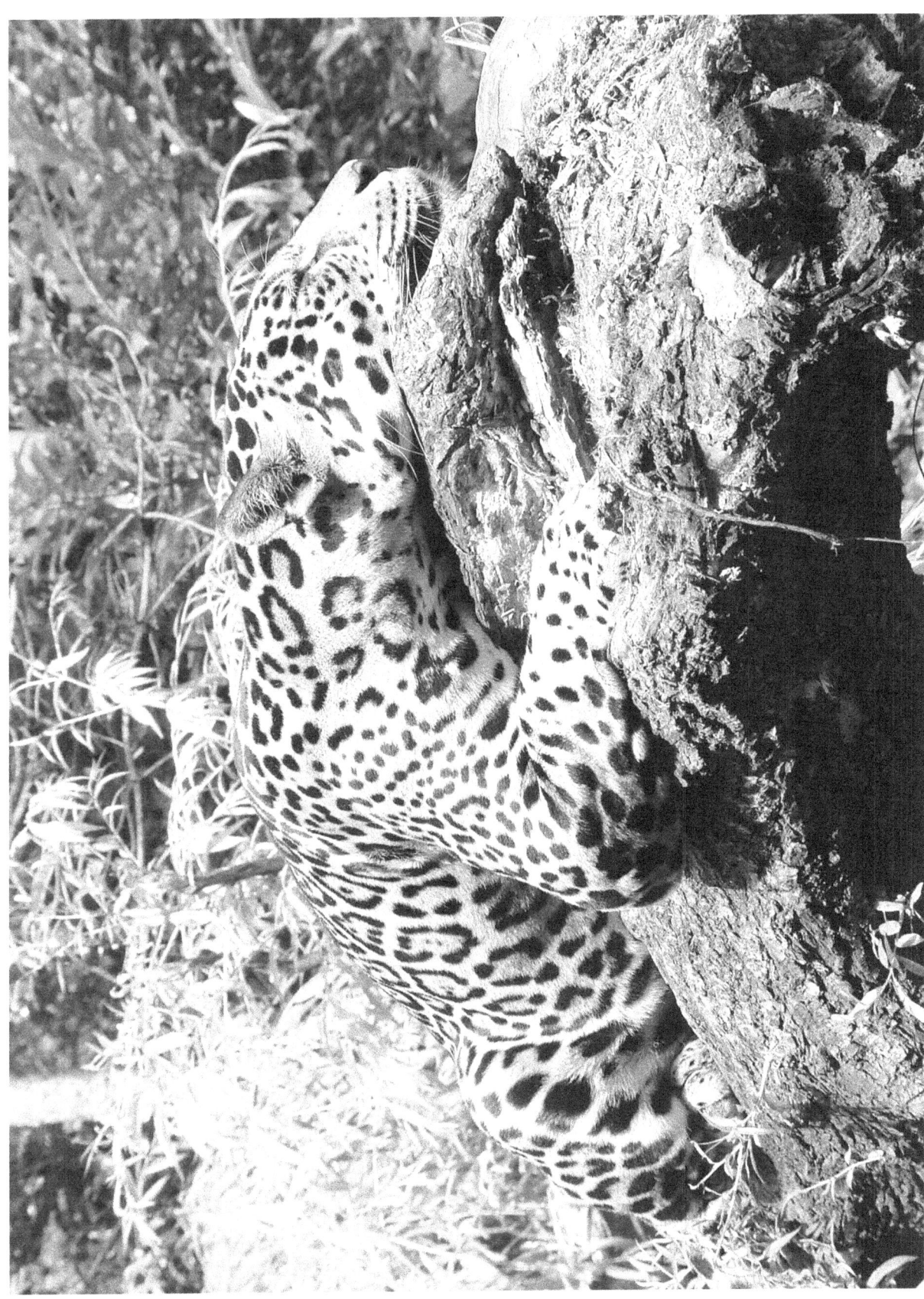

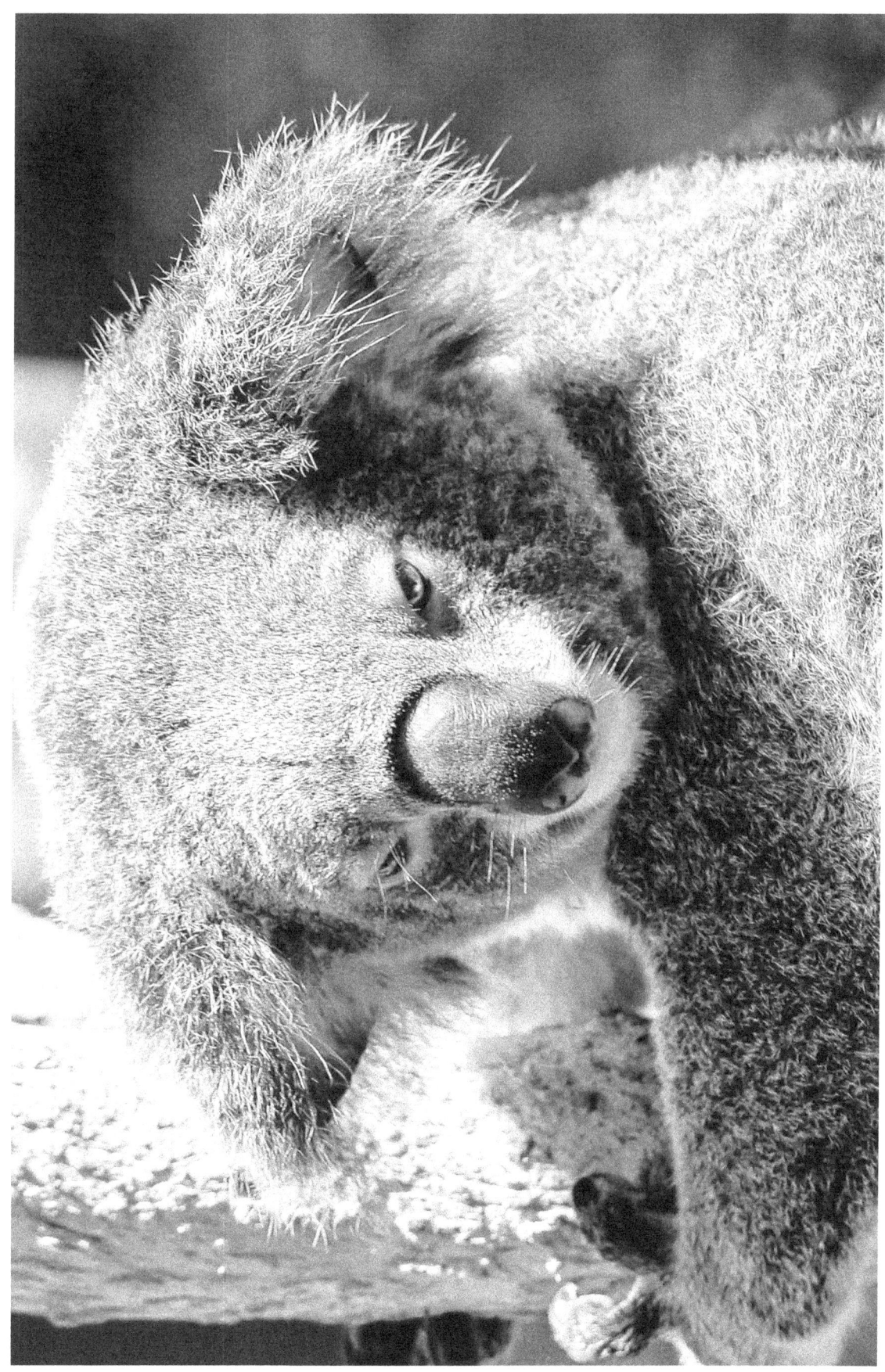

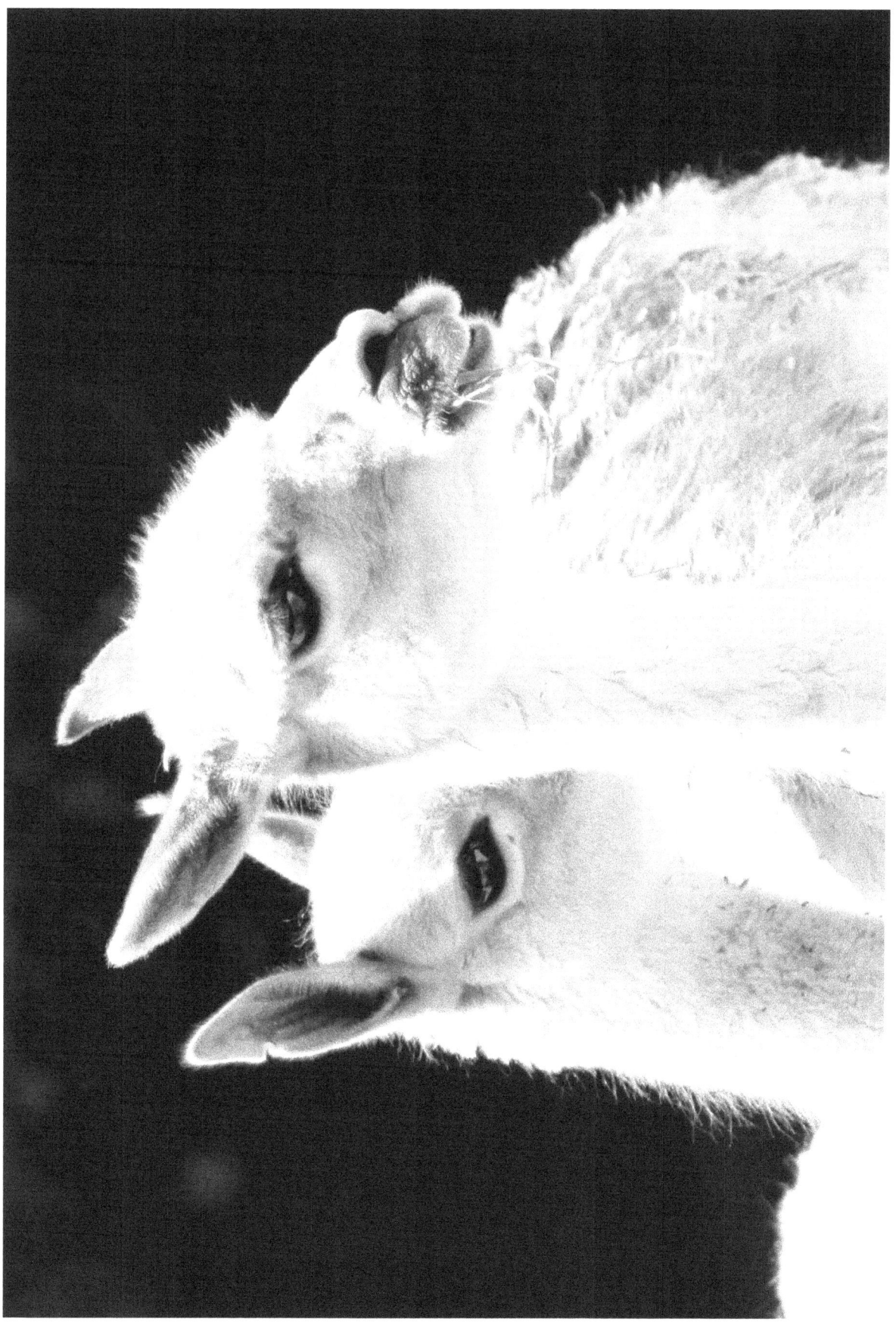

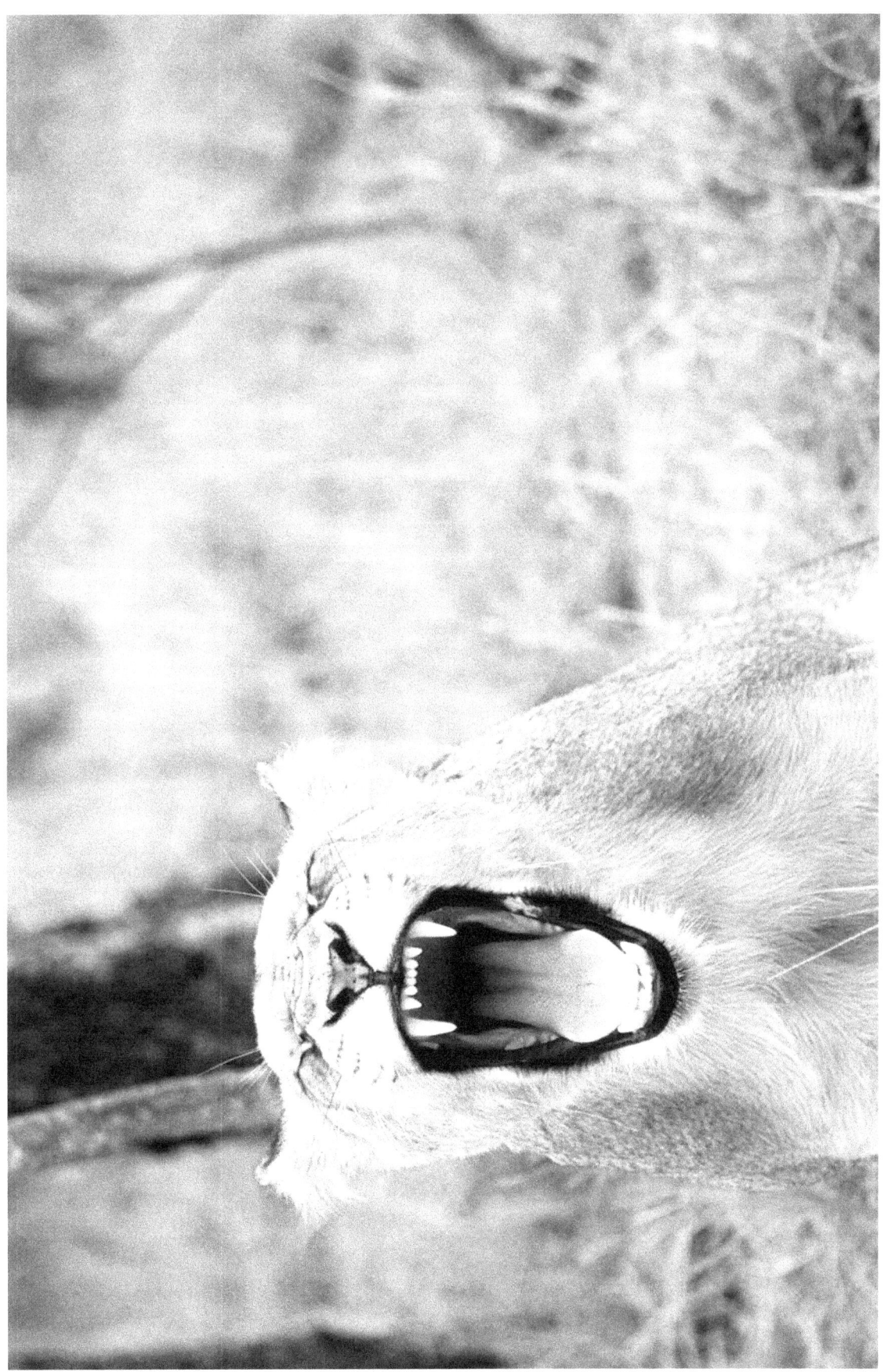

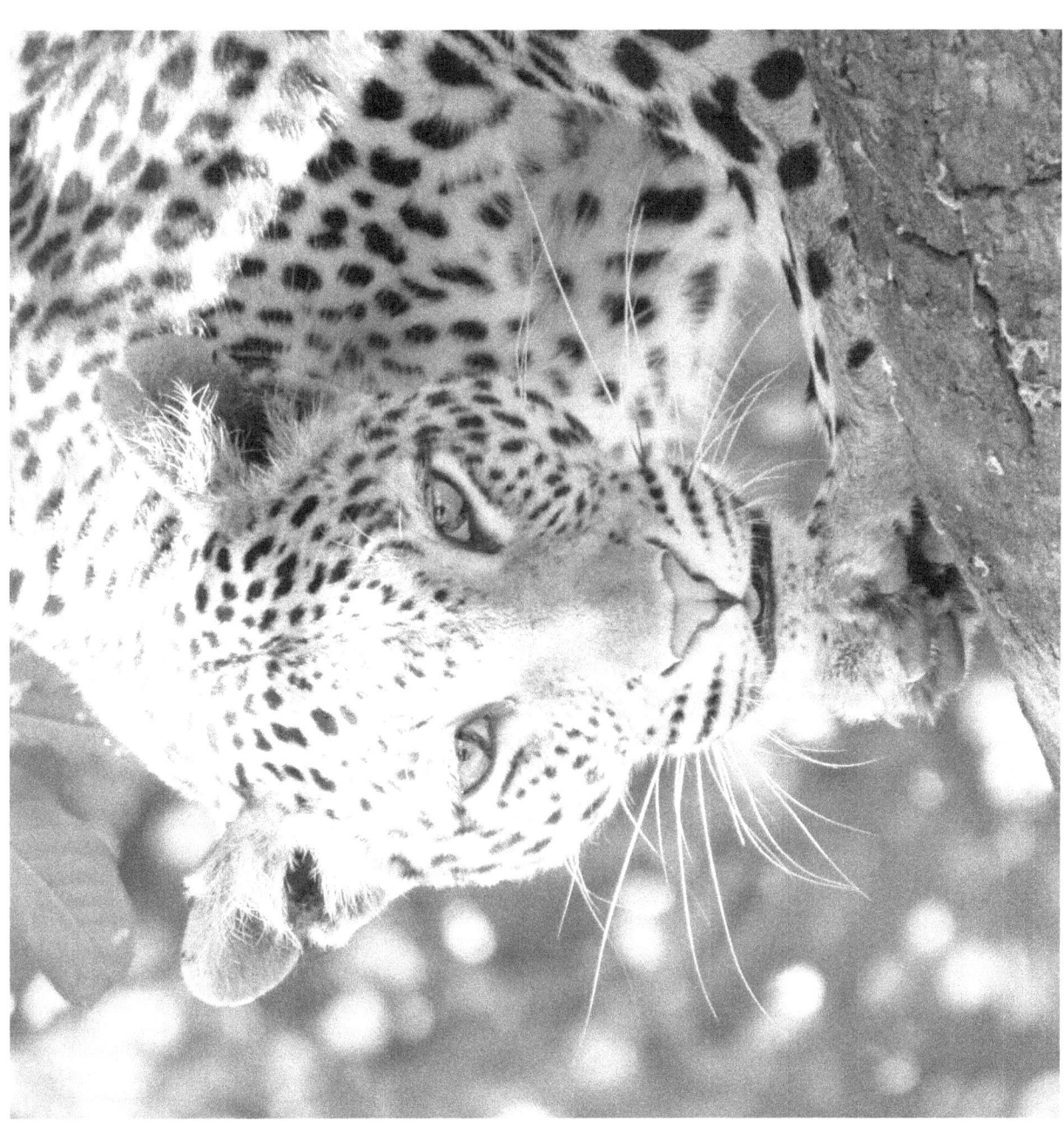

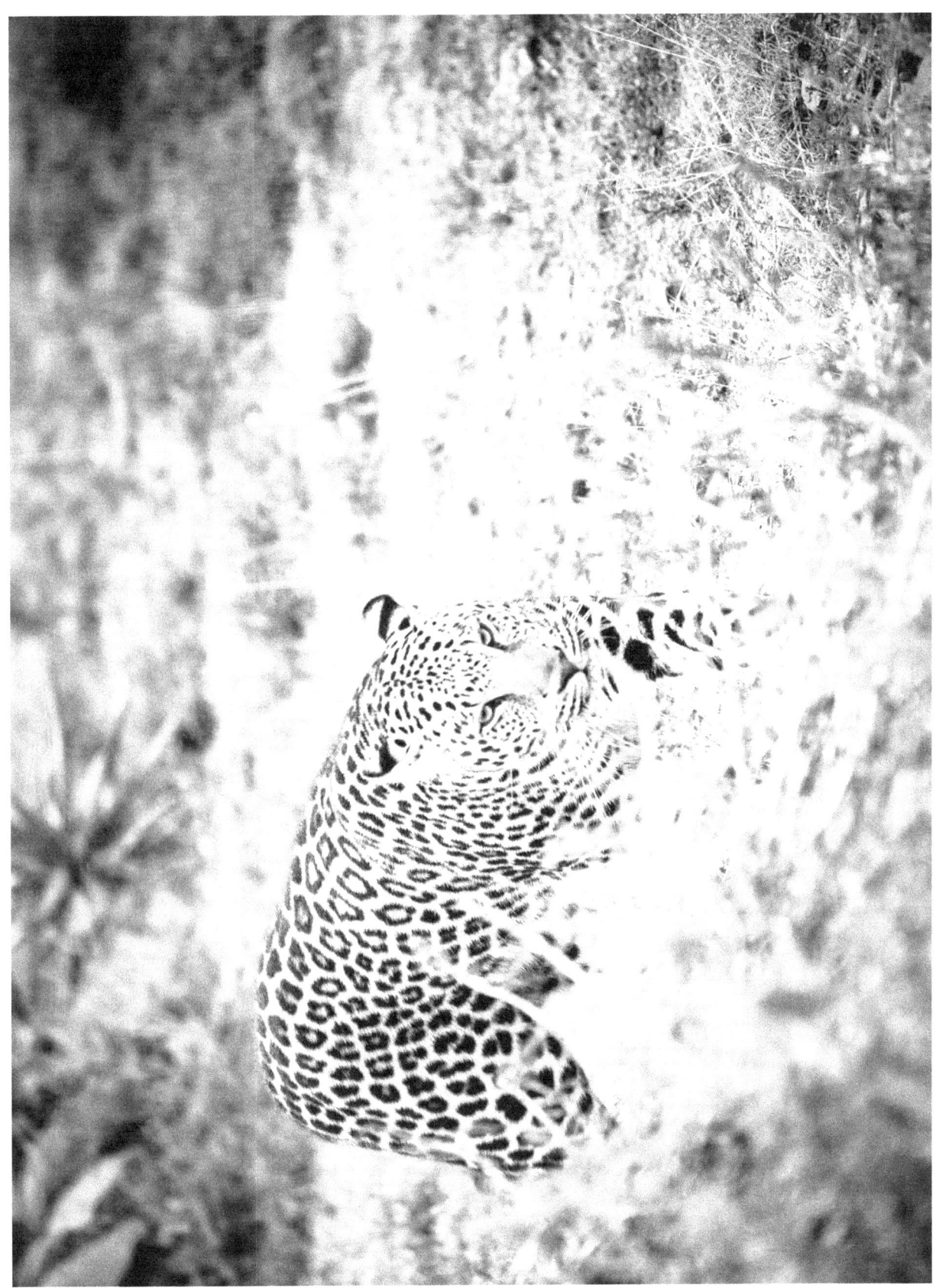

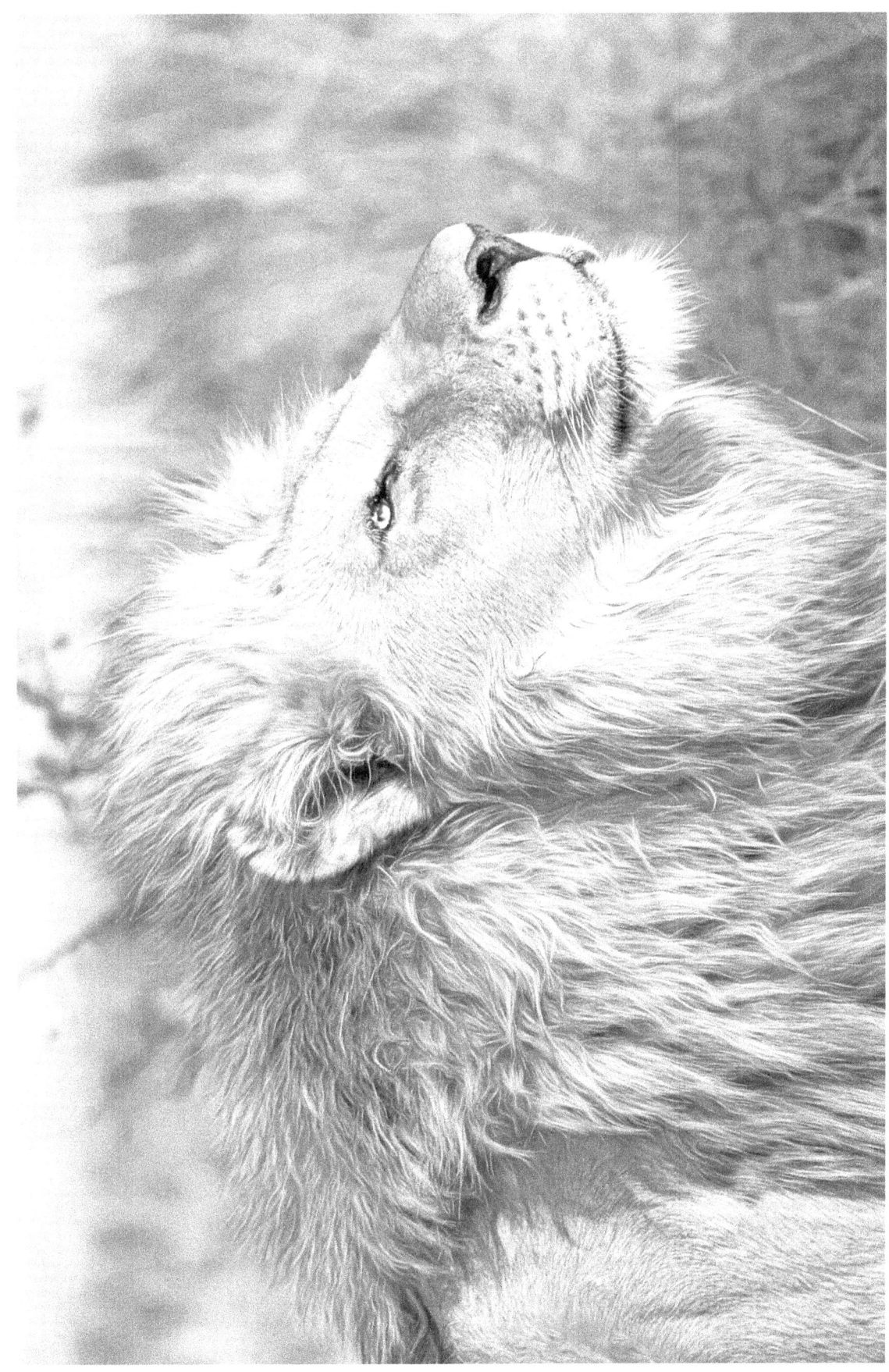

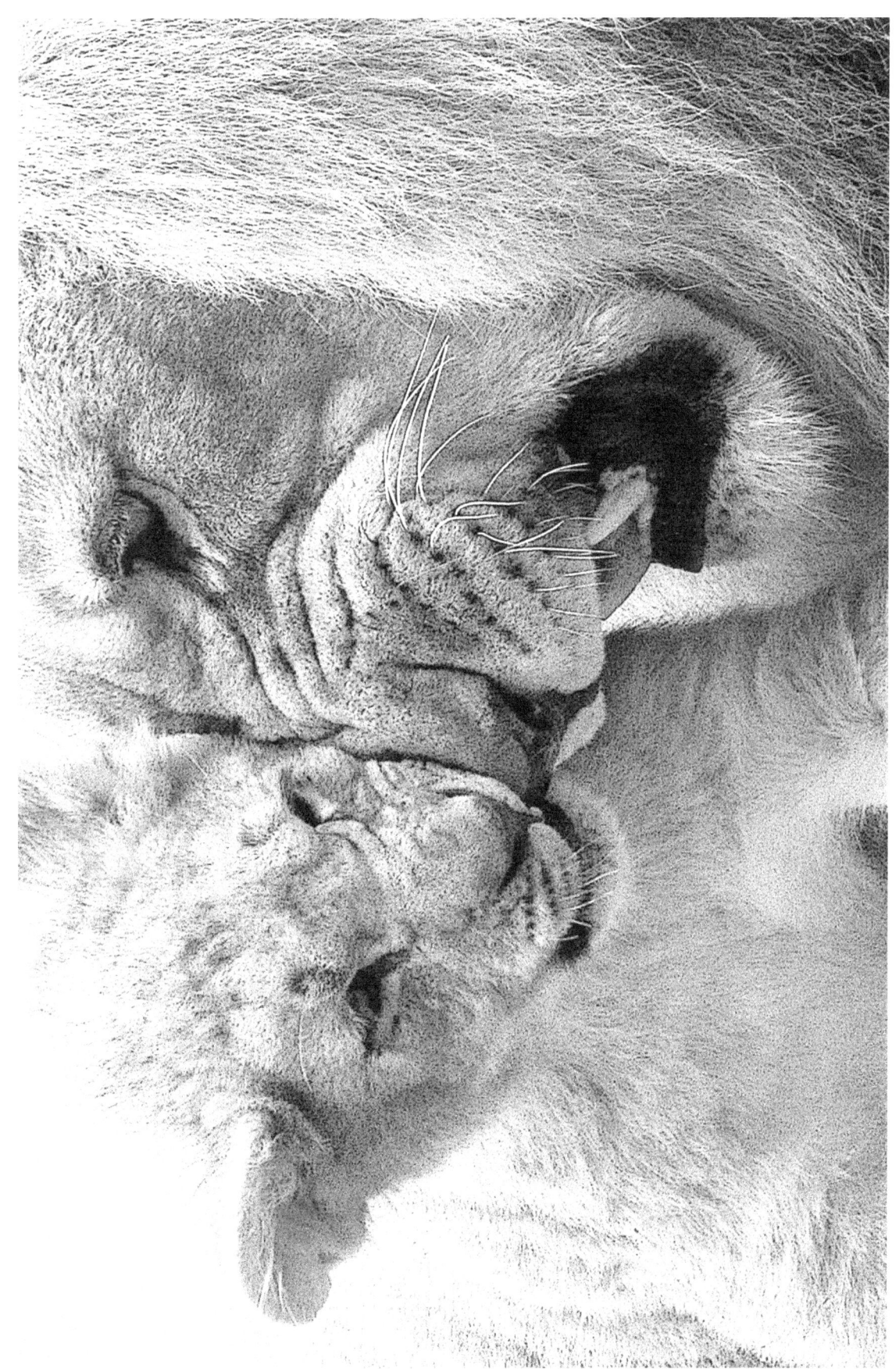

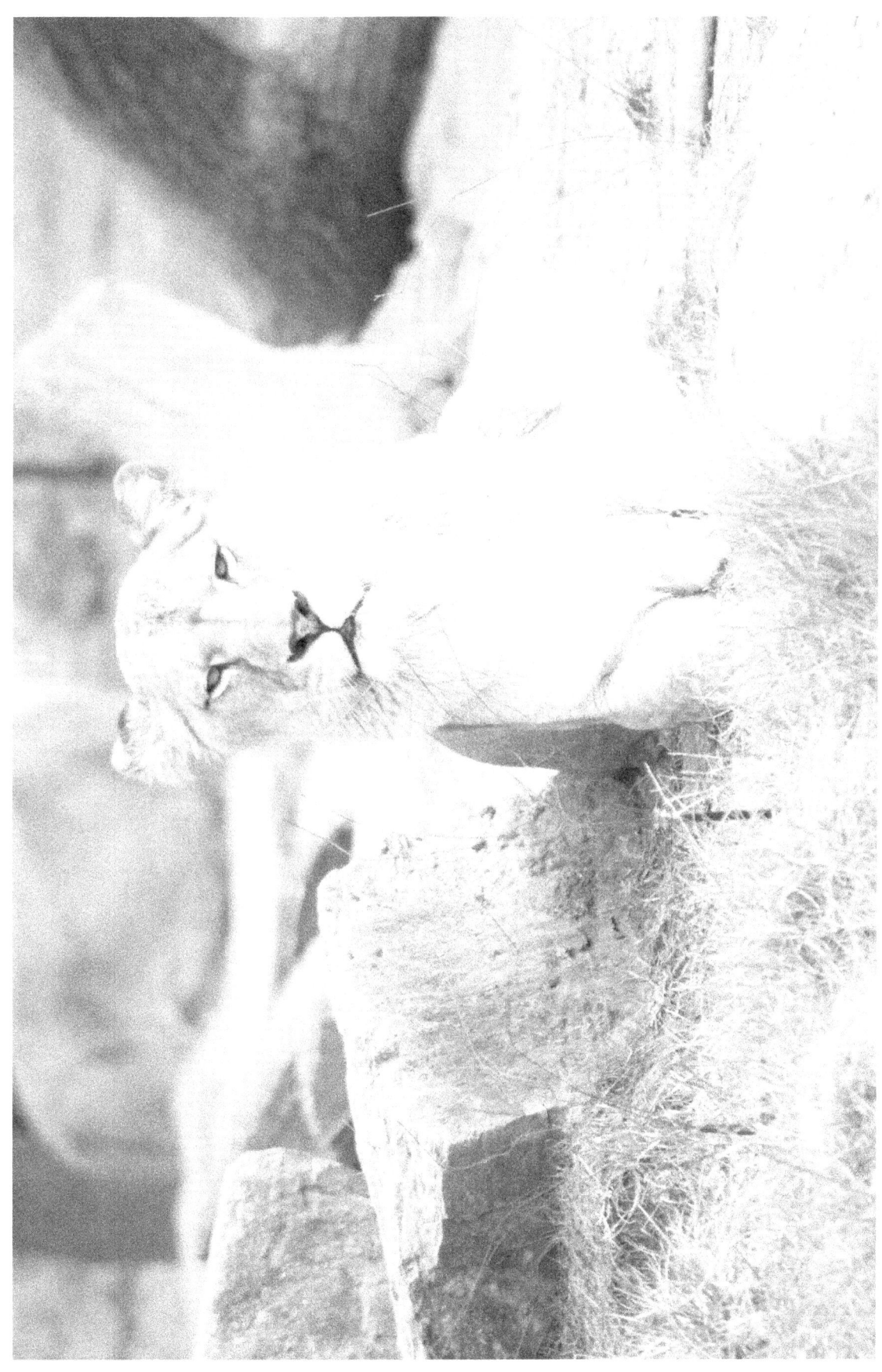

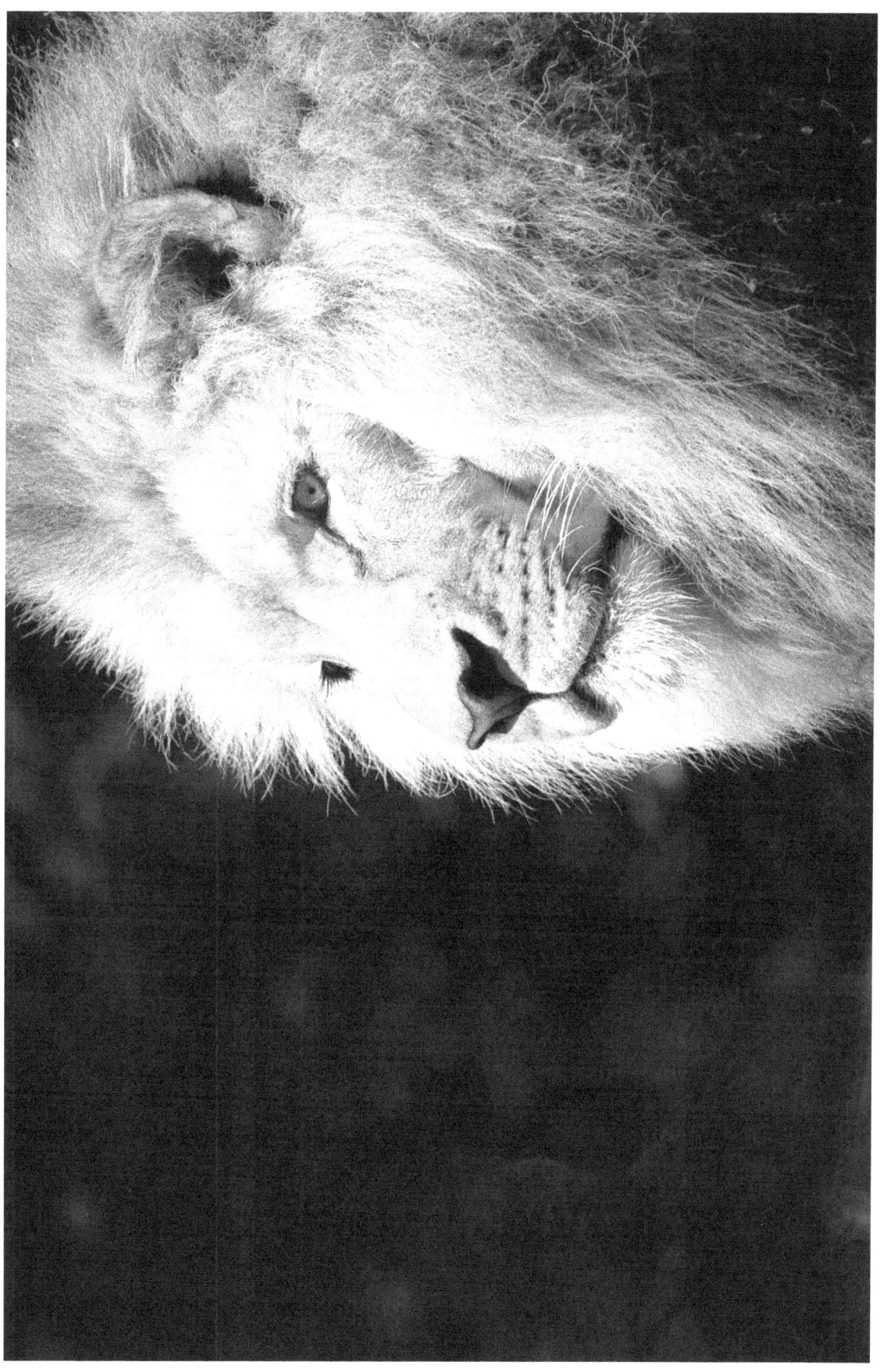

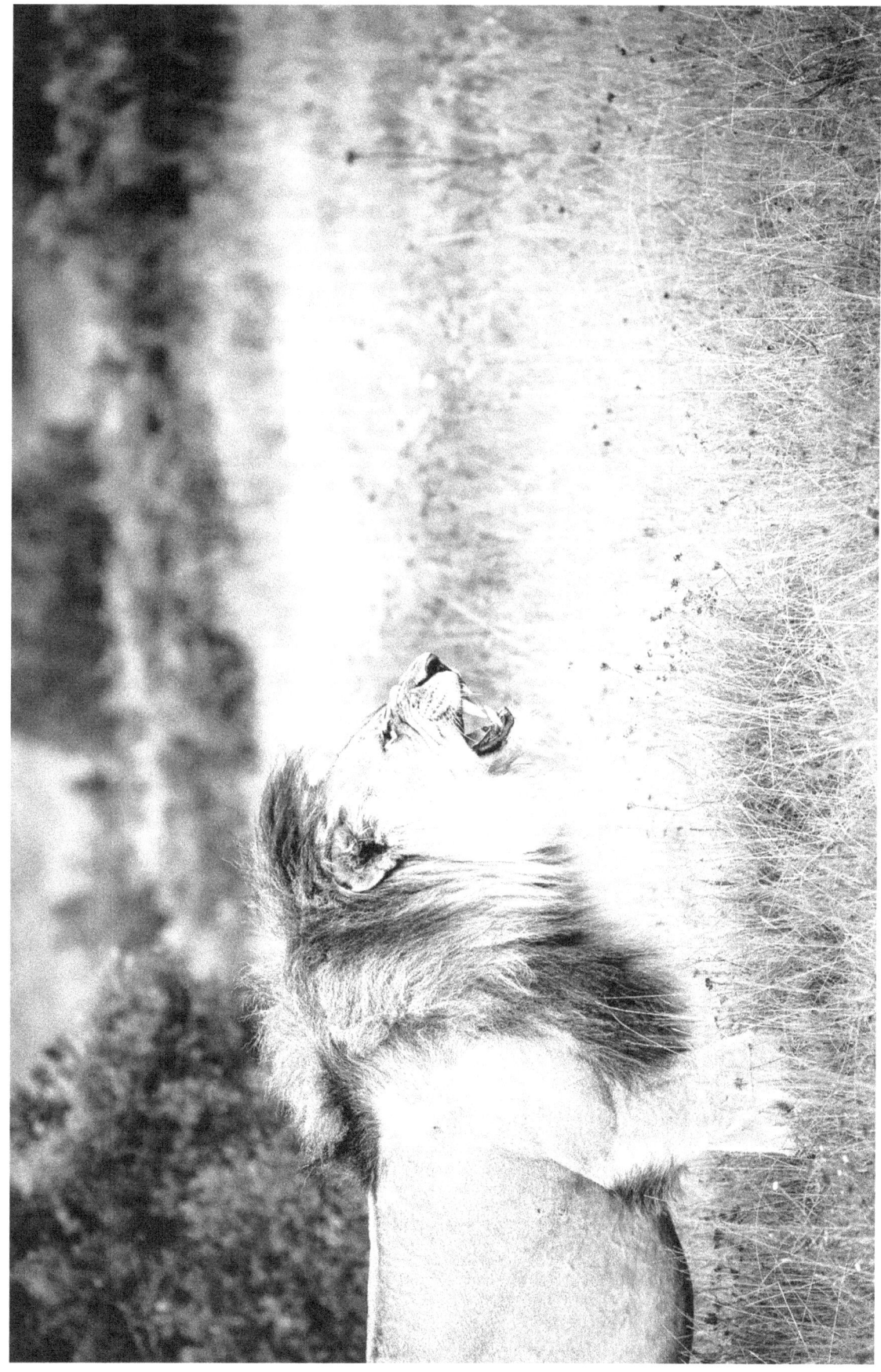

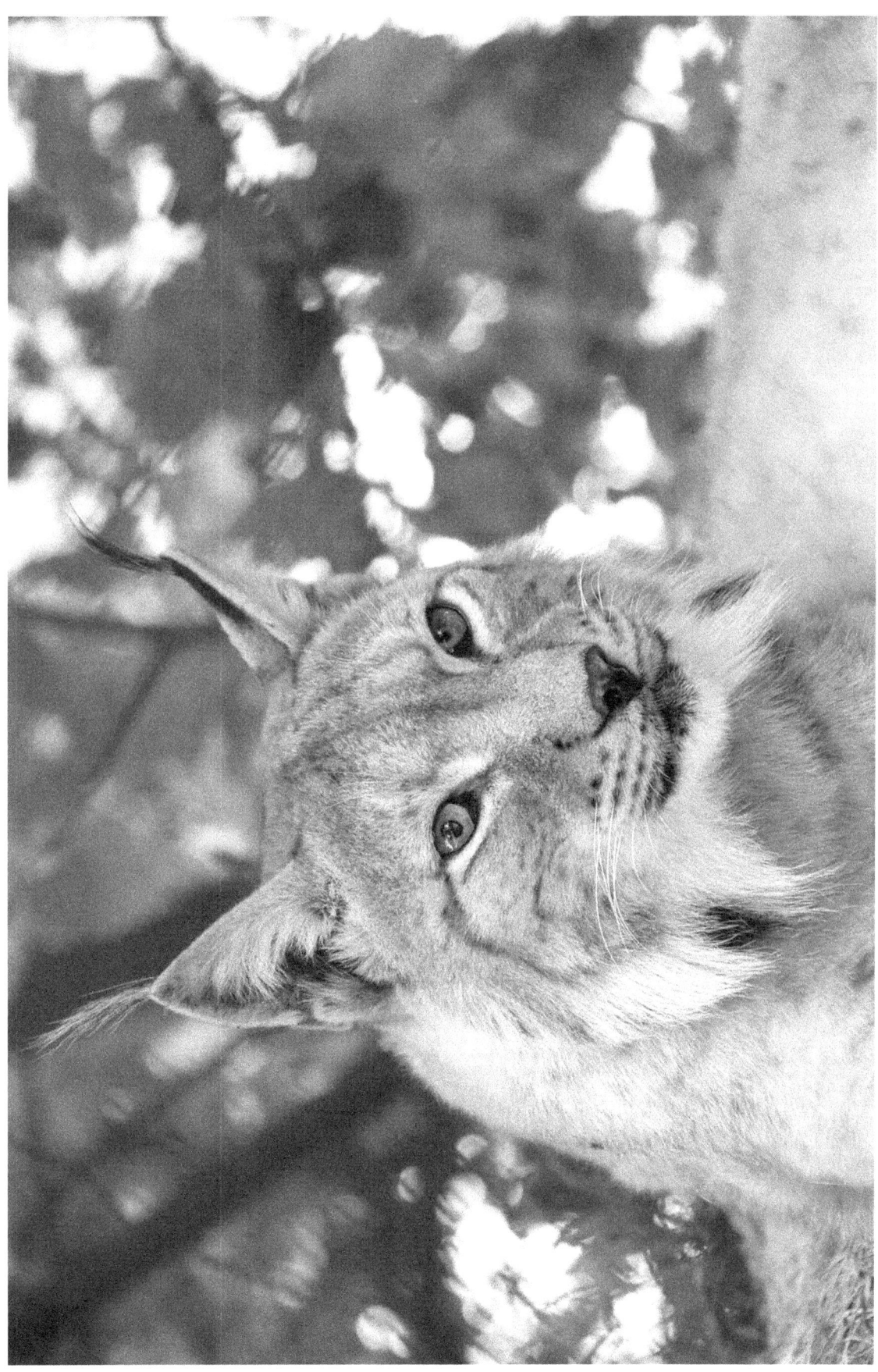

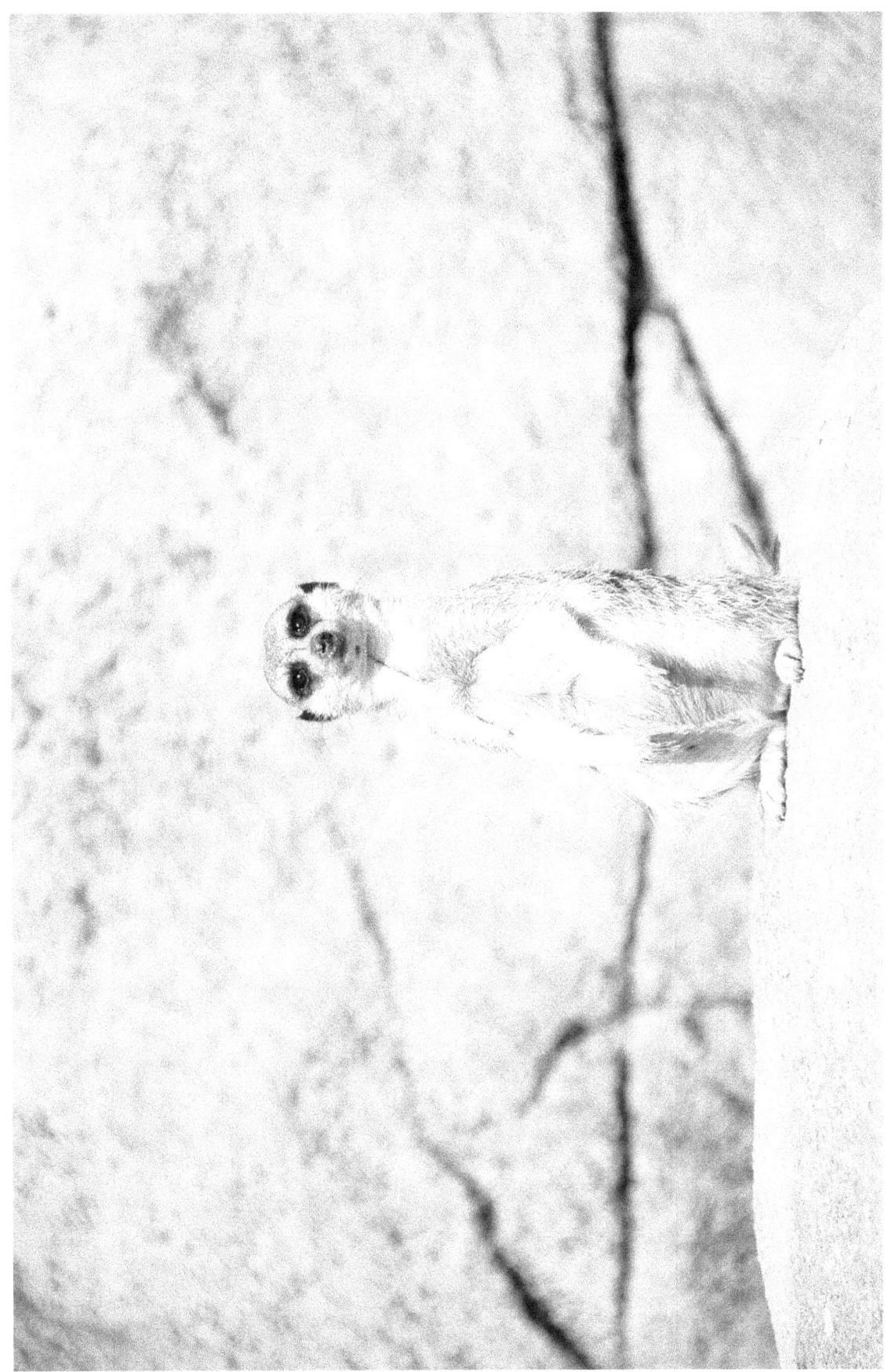

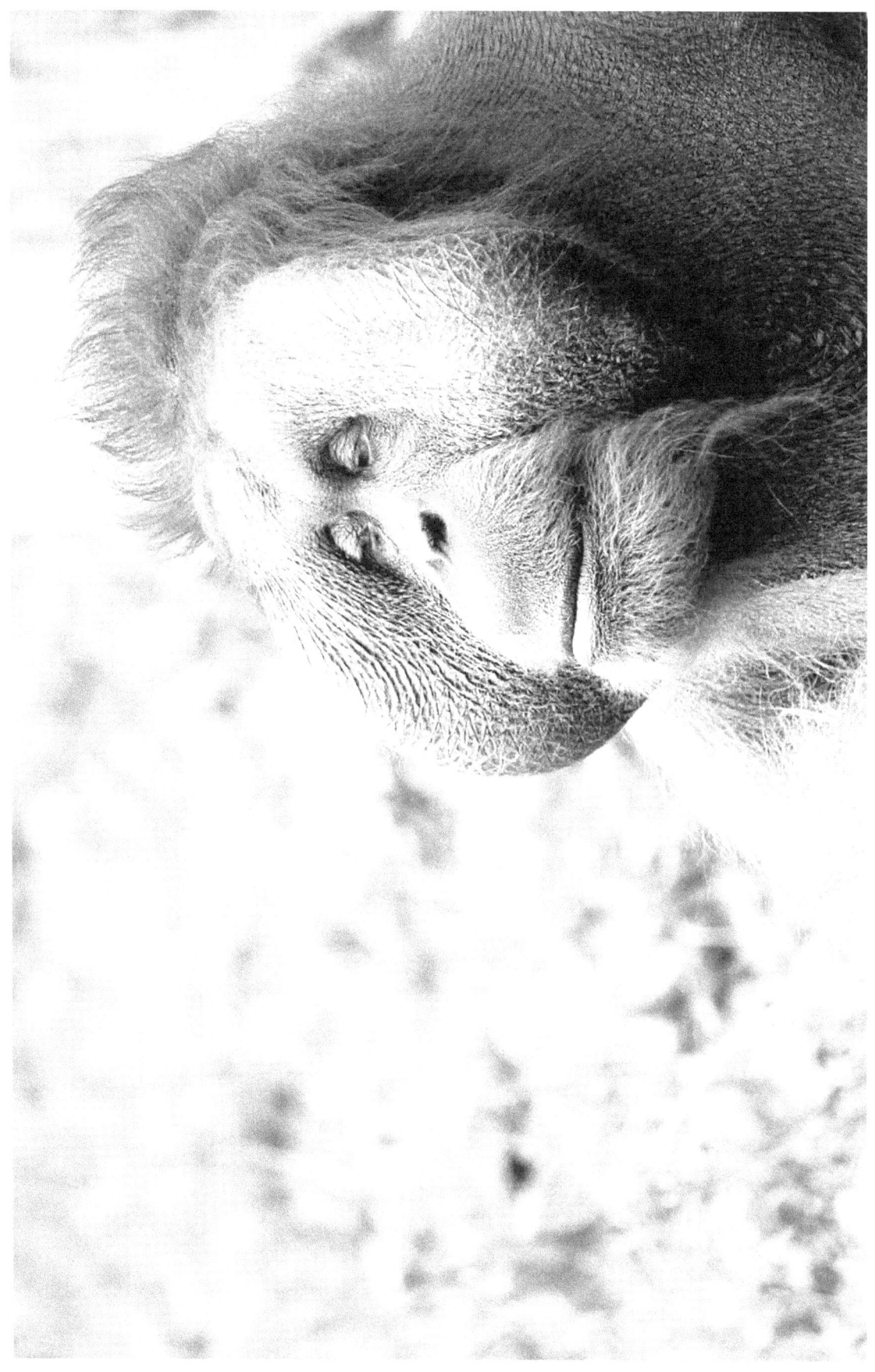

www.ingramcontent.com/pod-product-compliance
Lightning Source LLC
Chambersburg PA
CBHW080557190526
45169CB00007B/2807